THE KINGDOM HEALTH PLAN

ESTABLISHING THE KING'S KINGDOM ON EARTH

Forwarded by Imperial Nation Publishing

Syvonia McCoy

Contents

Introduction   ix

Chapter One   The Kingdom Covenant

Chapter Two   Understanding the Kingdom Realm of Life

Chapter Three   The Law of the Beasts

Chapter Four   Man's Health Plan

Chapter Five   Kingdom Food

Chapter six   Imperial Kingdom Health System

Preface

Now Enter Into Kingdom Healing

So many today are going through different health conditions within their earthly tabernacle until many have totally given up on walking in total health. Father has an awesome health plan for Kingdom Citizens, but we totally rely on man's health care plans and system. I am a firm believer that Yahweh is still healing today as he did yesterday. There's a cure for HIV AIDS and Cancer in G-d's Kingdom Health Plan. The health system of today has raised many eyebrows being that all medications given to treat a sickness, has a down side to it called "SIDE EFFECTS". I am a firm believer that the King Yahweh has a better health plan than that of man. I understand that it's through his power that doctors of today have obtained the knowledge they've obtained. I applaud them in every way, however, it is a great thing to know that the King had an original health plan designed for his people. The original plan was for us, as his children, to walk in total health! Being one of his Ambassadors of the Kingdom, I was petitioned to write this book concerning the King's health Plan. In reading this book, you are well on your way to increasing knowledge concerning the King's Plan for living a healthier lifestyle. I would like to touch and agree with you that upon the completion of this book, Kingdom Healing would be your portion. Please understand that you have a part to do as well in order to obtain your total healing. This book will help you to understand the King's Health Plan and how you can live in total Kingdom Health. It's totally up to you to apply the hidden treasures that are released in this book for you to walk in total health. I pray that this book would not just be another book on your book shelf, but a bible to you to assist you in reinventing your health. In anticipation and hope, may the King's Health Plan jolt you into divine health!

THE KINGDOM HEALTH PLAN

Dedicated to my mother Ilean, My handsome King, Melech Zabach Roy'El (Ken McCoy).

My babies always: Asia, Turra, Keetah , John, Li'Yah ,Semaj, Zion and the entie Imperial Nation Community. May each of you eat from the Kingdom Health Plan Forever.

Thy Kingdom Come, Thy will be done on earth as it is in heaven!

CHAPTER ONE

"THE COVENANT"

A **biblical covenant** is an agreement found in the bible between G-d and his people, the Israelites, in which G-d makes specific promises and demands.

The Mosaic Covenant, beginning in Exodus 19-24, contains the foundations of the Torah. In this covenant, God promises:

- To make the children of Israel His special possession among all people if they obey God and keep his covenant [Exo 19:5]
- To make the children of Israel a kingdom of priests and a holy nation[Exo 19:6]
- To give the children of Israel the Sabbath as the permanent sign of this covenant [Exo 31:12-17]

Before we go any further please understand that the definition of the word "Torah" is defined as G-d's teaching and Instructions. The Torah is the King's constitution, which are the first five books of the bible which comprises statutes and rules as to how to live a righteous set apart life-style which is pleasing to the King.

After the exodus of the Israelites out of Egypt, Moses went up on the Mount of Sinai to commune with Yahweh. While on the mount, Yahweh released a marriage covenant, which was the Torah, given to Moses for the children of Israel.

During this time that Yawheh released the covenant to Moses was during a feast called "Shavuots" (Pentecost). The Feast of Shavouts is a holy day which now commemorates the marriage covenant that Moses gave to the children of Israel fifty days after the Passover. The fifty days after the Passover count to Shavuots is called counting down of the Omer, the word omer is defined as "Sheaf".

Leviticus 23:15,16

[15] "'From the day after the Sabbath, the day you brought the sheaf (Barley) of the wave offering, count off seven full weeks. [16] Count off fifty days up to the day after the seventh Sabbath, and then present an offering of new grain to the LORD.

So many people today do not observe any of the seven feast found in Leviticus 23 nor count down the omer which Yahweh commanded. Because of this, many are missing out on a true personal relationship with ABBA. We must understand, in order to have a true personal relationship with the king, as well as to obtain all of the Kingdom's benefits, we must obey the king's commands. Everything the father does is in patterns! The scripture declares; "he's the same yesterday, today and forever more". The way he did things in Moses time, is the same thing he's doing in our time. He's an unchanging G-d!

Please understand that The Kingdom of G-d has seven days that we are to observe which was placed in the covenant, the torah, given to the children of Israel. These are the holy days of the King's Kingdom. Of course you know that everything the Kingdom of G-d does or have, Ha-Satan tries to duplicate.

The Seven Holy Days of the King's Kingdom are:

1. Passover (First Fruits)
2. Feast of Unleavened Bread
3. First Fruits (Yom Habbikurim)
4. Feast of Trumpets
5. Yom Kippur
6. Feast of Tabernacles (Succoth)
7. The Sabbath, Saturday, of each week is also called a holy day that father commanded us to reverence.

Leviticus 23:37

These are the feasts of the LORD, which ye shall proclaim to be holy convocations, to offer an offering made by fire unto the LORD, a burnt offering, and a meat offering, a sacrifice, and drink offerings, everything upon his day.

The counterfeit to the Holy Days of the King's Kingdom are:

1. Valentines Day (associated with greek pagan false gods)
2. Easter (counterfeit of the Passover)
3. St. Patricks Day (associated with greek pagan false gods)
4. Independence Day (man made day)
5. Christmas Day (no scriptural account as far as Christ's Birth being 25th of Dec.)

These are Pagan man made traditional Holi-Days of Ha'Satan's Kingdom which has nothing to do with the Kingdom of G-D.

Dan 7:25

And he shall speak *great* **words against the most High, and shall wear out the saints of the most High, and think to change times (FEAST DAYS) and laws: and they shall be given into his hand until a time and times and the dividing of time.**

A covenant is a promise; it's a vow that is kept throughout eternity, never to be broken. We as the children of Israel today must understand, in order to reap the benefits of the King's Kingdom, we must obey his commands and covenant that he originally intended for his children to follow.

CHAPTER TWO

"The Kingdom Realm of Life"

As King's Kids, we often times forget who we are! The reason we forget who we are is because we have exited into a realm other than the Kingdom Realm of Life.

Is. 53:8 He was taken from prison and from judgment: and who shall declare his generation, for he was cut off out of the land of the living: for the transgression of my people was he stricken.

The words "Cut Off" means exiled from Kingdom Living and benefits. When we walk against the grain of the King's commands we are cut off from the Kingdom Realm of Life. Once we are cut off, we enter into another realm called the realm of death. In the realm of death, everything in our lives begins to deteriorate. Our health, finances, spirituality, etc all began to wither away. G-d original plan was for us to have life and have it more abundantly. Today we can have life and it more abundantly if we return to him and seek the Kingdom to its entirety. He wants us to walk in the realm of life, this is the reason he gave Moses the Kingdom Covenant as a measuring tool for us to measure our lifestyle accordingly. When we go against or disobey what has been written, we are cut off from that realm. Many do not understand that in the covenant or the constitution given to Moses, it has a blue print for our everyday living. Because of Moses misrepresentation of the father, he did not enter into the promise land, he was cut off, and this allows us to see that we have a part to do in order to walk in the realm of life.

Numbers 20:7-12

[7]And the LORD spake unto Moses, saying, [8]Take the rod, and gather thou the assembly together, thou, and Aaron thy brother, and speak ye unto the rock before their eyes; and it shall give forth his water, and thou shalt bring forth to them water out of the rock: so thou shalt give the congregation and their beasts drink.

⁹And Moses took the rod from before the LORD, as he commanded him. ¹⁰And Moses and Aaron gathered the congregation together before the rock, and he said unto them, Hear now, ye rebels; must we fetch you water out of this rock? ¹¹And Moses lifted up his hand, and with his rod he smote the rock twice: and the water came out abundantly, and the congregation drank, and their beasts also. ¹²And the LORD spake unto Moses and Aaron, Because ye believed me not, to sanctify me in the eyes of the children of Israel, therefore ye shall not bring this congregation into the land which I have given them.

Many of us do not like to associate our choices with why we go through in our lives. What many do not understand is that the Kingdom of G-D has a reap and sow system. For an example if you sow eating junk food, you will reap a harvest of having bad health which will cut you off from the realm of life. Continually eating the wrong foods will keep us in the realm of death, our health will continue to deteriorate because we are not eating the foods found in the covenant. It's sad to say that we are living in a toxic world where our atmosphere is highly sedated with toxic waste. Pesticides and chemical injections has been a thing of today which is implemented in our daily food intake. Ha-Satan has a very crafty way of infecting people with health issues because he knows many do not understand the covenant which was given to Moses. Later in this book you will find out the foods that will keep you in the realm of life and which foods cut you off from the King's Health Plan.

Return Back to the King!

Chapter Three

"The Laws of the Beasts"

Leviticus 11:46-47

⁴⁶This is the law of the beasts, and of the fowl, and of every living creature that moveth in the waters, and of every creature that creepeth upon the earth ⁴⁷To make a difference between the unclean and the clean, and between the beast that may be eaten and the beast that may not be eaten.

In this chapter you will explore the foods in the covenant given to Moses from Yahweh on the Mount of Sinai. As declared in Leviticus 11, we must understand the difference between clean and unclean. The clean beasts of the field are what we are to eat. Eating clean will keep us from experiencing health issues such as High blood pressure, diabetes, headaches, etc.. the list goes on and on. When we eat of the unclean beast, this cut us off from the realm of Kingdom Life. This is the reason why we began experiencing health issues because when we eat unclean things, we automatically began to walk in the realm of Death. We began to reap the seeds sown concerning "The Laws of the Beasts"

Leviticus 7:21

Moreover the soul that shall touch any unclean thing, as the uncleanness of man, or any unclean beast, or any abominable unclean thing, and eat of the flesh of the sacrifice of peace offerings, which pertain unto the LORD, even that soul shall be cut off from his people.

Have you ever went into a restaurant and ordered a steak medium rare, do you know that this is an unclean thing to do? Abba commanded us in the torah not to eat or drink blood. G-d says that the life is in the blood. It carries away various toxins, viruses and bacteria for elimination. Let's see what the scripture says concerning this:

Leviticus 7:26-27

 Moreover ye shall eat no manner of blood, whether it be of fowl or of beast, in any of your dwellings. ²⁷Whatsoever soul it be that eateth any manner of blood, even that soul shall be cut off from his people.

We are also commanded not to eat the fat of a beast. We all are guilty in this; many of our ancestors couldn't cook a pot of fresh collards without throwing in a piece of fatback bacon! What most of us doesn't realize is that animals and humans store poisons and viruses in their fat. When people eat fat, they are ingesting additional poisons.

Our traditions have caused many of us to have habits that we are finding so much difficult to break this day. Some of you may be asking what does the bible says concerning the fat of a beast. Well let's go to the scripture and find out.

Leviticus 7:23

Speak unto the children of Israel, saying, Ye shall eat no manner of fat, of ox, or of sheep, or of goat

Scripture tells us in Leviticus 7:25 if we eat the fat of an animal we will surely be cut off from the Kingdom Health Plan.

²⁵For whosoever eateth the fat of the beast, of which men offer an offering made by fire unto the LORD, even the soul that eateth it shall be cut off from his people.

When we go against what the King commanded, we go against his Kingdom Health Plan. Therefore, we are no longer covered under the King's hand. I don't know about you, but I find this to be a dangerous place to be! This is the reason sickness and disease has infiltrated our lives because we are not being obedient to the torah. I'm so glad that it's not too late to "TESHUVAH" a Hebrew word for Return and Repent. When we return and repent to Yahweh he will restore us back to the original Kingdom Plan for our life. It's not by accident that you are reading this book, it's your season to return to him and embrace the covenant concerning your diet. In doing this, your health is on its way to total recovery!

Which Animals Does the Bible Designate as 'Clean' and 'Unclean'?

God reveals which animals—including fish and birds—are suitable and unsuitable for human consumption in Leviticus 11 and Deuteronomy 14.

Although the lists aren't exhaustive, He reveals guidelines for recognizing animals that are acceptable for food.

God states that cud-chewing animals with split hooves can be eaten

Leviticus: 11:3 Whatsoever parteth the hoof, and is clovenfooted, and cheweth the cud, among the beasts, that shall ye eat.;

Deuteronomy: 14:6 And every beast that parteth the hoof, and cleaveth the cleft into two claws, and cheweth the cud among the beasts, that ye shall eat.). These specifically include the cattle, sheep, goat, deer and gazelle families

Deuteronomy: 14:4-5 These are the beasts which ye shall eat: the ox, the sheep, and the goat, The hart, and the roebuck, and the fallow deer, and the wild goat, and the pygarg, and the wild ox, and the chamois.). He also lists such animals as camels, rabbits and pigs as being unclean, or unfit to eat

Leviticus: 11:4-8 Nevertheless these shall ye not eat of them that <u>chew the cud</u>, or of them that divide the hoof: as the camel, because he cheweth the cud, but divideth not the hoof; he is unclean unto you. And the coney, because he cheweth the cud, but divideth not the hoof; he is unclean unto you. And the hare, because he cheweth the cud, but divideth not the hoof; he is unclean unto you. And the swine, though he divide the hoof, and be clovenfooted, yet he cheweth not the cud; he is unclean to you. Of their flesh shall ye not eat, and their carcase shall ye not touch; they are unclean to you.

He later lists such "creeping things" as moles, mice and lizards as unfit to eat (verses 29-31), as well as four-footed animals with paws (cats, dogs, bears, lions, tigers, etc.) as unclean (verse 27).

He tells us that salt and freshwater fish with fins and scales may be eaten (verses 9-12), but water creatures without those characteristics (catfish, lobsters, crabs, shrimp, mussels, clams, oysters, squid, octopi, etc.) should not be eaten.

God also lists birds and other flying creatures that are unclean for consumption (verses 13-19). He identifies carrion eaters and birds of prey as unclean, plus ostriches, storks, herons and bats.

Birds such as chickens, turkeys and pheasants are not on the unclean list and therefore can be eaten. Insects, with the exception of locusts, crickets and grasshoppers, are listed as unclean (verses 20-23).

Why does G-d identify some animals as suitable for human consumption and others as unsuitable? G-d didn't give laws to arbitrarily assert control over people. He gave His laws (including those of which meats are clean or unclean) "that it might be well" with those who seek to obey Him.

Deuteronomy:5:29 that there were such an heart in them, that they would fear me, and keep all my commandments always, that it might be well with them, and with their children for ever

Although G-d did not reveal the specific reasons some animals may be eaten and others must be avoided, we can make generalized conclusions based on the animals included in the two categories. In listing the animals that should not be eaten, G-d forbids the consumption of scavengers and carrion eaters, which devour other animals for their food.

Animals such as pigs, bears, vultures and raptors can eat (and thrive) on decaying flesh. Predatory animals such as wolves, lions, leopards and cheetahs most often prey on the weakest (and at times the diseased) in animal herds.

When it comes to sea creatures, bottom dwellers such as lobsters and crabs scavenge for dead animals on the sea floor. Shellfish such as oysters, clams and mussels similarly consume decaying organic matter that sinks to the sea floor, including sewage, these are called the cleaners of the sea floor.

A common denominator of many of the animals G-d designates as unclean is that they routinely eat flesh that would sicken or kill human beings. When we eat such animals, we partake of a food chain that includes things harmful to people.

Eating against what the King has declared will cause you to be "cut off" from the Kingdom Health Plan.

Clean Animals

Mammals That Chew the Cud and Part the Hoof

Antelope
Bison (buffalo)
Caribou
Cattle (beef, veal)
Deer (venison)
Elk
Gazelle
Giraffe
Goat
Hart
Ibex
Moose
Ox
Reindeer
Sheep (lamb, mutton)

Fish With Fins and Scales

Anchovy
Barracuda
Bass
Black pomfret (or monchong)
Bluefish
Bluegill
Carp
Cod
Crappie
Drum
Flounder
Grouper
Grunt
Haddock
Hake
Halibut
Hardhead
Herring (or alewife)
Kingfish
Mackerel (or corbia)
Mahimahi (or dorado, dolphinfish [not to be confused with the mammal dolphin])
Minnow
Mullet
Perch (or bream)
Pike (or pickerel or jack)
Pollack (or pollock or Boston bluefish)
Rockfish
Salmon
Sardine (or pilchard)
Shad
Silver hake (or whiting)
Smelt (or frost fish or ice fish)
Snapper (or ebu, jobfish, lehi, onaga, opakapaka or uku)
Sole
Steelhead
Sucker
Sunfish
Tarpon
Trout (or weakfish)
Tuna (or ahi, aku, albacore, bonito or tombo)
Turbot (except European turbot)
Whitefish

Unclean Animals

Animals With Unclean Characteristics

Swine

Boar
Peccary
Pig (hog, bacon, ham, lard, pork, most sausage and pepperoni)

Canines

Coyote
Dog
Fox
Hyena
Jackal
Wolf

Felines

Cat
Cheetah
Leopard
Lion
Panther
Tiger

Equines

Donkey (ass)
Horse
Mule
Onager
Zebra (quagga)

Other

Armadillo
Badger
Bat
Bear
Beaver
Groundhog
Hippopotamus
Kangaroo
Llama (alpaca, vicuña)
Mole
Monkey
Mouse
Muskrat
Opossum
Porcupine
Rabbit (hare)
Raccoon
Rat
Rhinoceros
Skunk
Slug
Snail (escargot)
Squirrel
Wallaby
Weasel
Wolverine
Worm
All insects except some in the locust family

Marine Animals Without Fins and Scales

Fish

Bullhead
Catfish
Eel
European Turbot
Marlin
Paddlefish
Shark
Stickleback
Squid
Sturgeon (includes most

Shellfish

Abalone
Clam
Conch
Crab
Crayfish (crawfish, crawdad)
Lobster
Mussel
Oyster
Scallop
Shrimp (prawn)

Soft body

Cuttlefish
Jellyfish
Limpet
Octopus
Squid (calamari)

Sea mammals

Dolphin
Otter
Porpoise
Seal
Walrus
Whale

Birds of Prey, Scavengers and Others

Albatross
Bittern
Buzzard
Condor
Coot
Cormorant
Crane
Crow

Cuckoo

15 The Imperial Kingdom Health Plan

Camel	caviar)		Eagle
Elephant		Swordfish	Flamingo
Gorilla			

YOU SHALL BE HOLY

God says in Leviticus 19:2, "You shall be holy: for I, the Lord your God, am holy."

Eating anything unclean is the opposite of holy which is termed "Defile". When you eat these things you are defiling your temple allowing the realm of death to be your portion.

The animals above do not have a filtering system, let's take for an example an alligator, or any of the above animals listed on the unclean chart, if any of these animals were to consume something or someone with HIV these animals have no way of filtering this disease from its system. When we eat these animals we are walking in total disobedience to the Kingdom's Health Plan, these animals defiles the temple.

PHYSICAL CURSES FOR DISOBEDIENCE

And what about the actual diseases many of unclean animals carry, of which trichinosis is the most commonly known? Physical curses promised to ancient Israel for disobedience to the laws that God gave to them.

Deuteronomy 28:22 "The Lord shall smite you a consumption, and a fever and with an inflammation, and with an extreme burning..."Verses 27-28 - "The Lord shall smite you with the botch of Egypt, and with the emerods, and with the scab, with the itch whereof you cannot be healed, Lord shall smite you with madness, and blind and astonishment of heart." Verse 35 - "The Lord shall smite you in the knees, and in the legs with a sore botch that cannot be healed from the sole of your foot unto the top of your head."

What are the diseases mentioned here? Cancer, heart disease, rheumatism, arthritis, and other degenerative diseases among the curses described.

Scavengers

Most of the creatures identified as unclean are actually scavengers. God designed them to be "garbage collectors"—a kind of "environmental cleanup crew." These scavengers are capable of ingesting and processing tremendous amounts of poison and waste in short periods of time.

Some scavengers, such as catfish, crabs and lobsters, are bottom-feeders. Others, like vultures and crows, eat dead, rotting flesh. This assists in the breakdown of organic matter and bacteria, so that they do not remain toxic or dangerous to the environment.

Pigs can eat rattlesnakes and have often been used to clear areas where golf courses are planned. Anything a pig eats turns to flesh in approximately six hours. Cows require twenty-four or more. Hogs actually have specially designed pus ducts located above their hooves to regularly drain poisons from their bodies. They carry a number of viruses and diseases, including trichina worms, which, if ingested by humans, can cause the painful and sometimes fatal disease known as *Trichinosis*. Also, pig flesh is high in cholesterol, which is one of the first things doctors tell patients with coronary artery disease to avoid in their diets.

Misguided mankind has domesticated pigs for food and put them in pigsties, literally forcing them to wallow in their own filth. This can cause their pus ducts to become plugged. Thus, those people who eat them ingest even more poison than God ever intended even filthy pigs to carry!

While many scavengers are far from beautiful, these creatures actually demonstrate, in their own way, the perfect planning and creative genius of God!

Romans 14:14 plainly state that *nothing is unclean of itself?*

Our English translations do, but the Greek, in which it was originally written, does not! The Greek word used here is *koinon*. It appears three times within this one verse and it does *not* mean *unclean*. It should be translated "common." This is the often-used biblical term that is the equivalent of *defiled*. Recall Matthew 15 and Mark 7. In those accounts, the similar word, *koinos,* is consistently translated as a form of *defile*.

This is also one of the two words used in Acts 10:14 to relate what Peter said during his vision. There, it is correctly translated to show that he had never eaten anything *common* (or unclean). The Greek word for *unclean* is *akatharton*. These two words do *not* have the same meaning. *Akatharton* means *unclean* and is used to distinguish clean creatures from unclean creatures. *Koinon* means *common*, and should have been so translated.

It is interesting to note that every translator and reviser, almost without exception, from A.D. 1611 forward, mistranslated this word as "unclean" in Romans 14:14. Somehow they always managed to get it right *everywhere else* in the New Testament. The context has *nothing at all* to do with *the distinction* between clean and unclean meat.

Why be concerned about something being *common*, if it is already *unclean*? What would be the difference?

Even before the Israelites were forbidden to eat unclean animals, they were prohibited from eating any animal that was torn by beasts in the field (Ex. 22:31). If an Israelite ate the flesh of any clean animal, which had died of itself (this was not be permissible—Deut. 14:21), that *person* was "unclean" until evening (Lev. 11:40). It means he was *defiled*. (This was the sort of defiling which does not come about by eating with unwashed hands!)

No priest was permitted to defile himself by eating animals that died naturally or were torn by beasts (Lev. 22:7). In Romans 14:14, Paul was teaching that the "Jewish" concept of meats sometimes being *common* or defiled, was not an intrinsic property of the meat itself, but was a matter of perception and conscience.

As well as being vital to all who were in Rome (Rom. 1:7), this teaching was also important to the Church at Corinth.

Chapter Four

"Man's Health Plan"

Today, Americans spend almost 20 cents of every dollar managing disease – diabetes, allergies, asthma, cancer, obesity - and only 10 cents of every dollar on food. The jury is still out on what exactly may be causing all of these epidemics, but genetics don't change that quickly, the environment does.

We all know eating clean helps us look and feel our best, but there is another great reason to upgrade your life style change: a Kingdom healthy diet can save you a ton of money on health care costs.

Over the past decade, health insurance rates have skyrocketed. In the last two years, monthly premiums in the United States were 131% higher than they were in 2000, according to the **Kaiser Family Foundation**. This is largely due to the high cost of treating diseases related to unhealthy diets. According to **a recent study** by the U.S. Centers for Disease Control and Prevention, the Agency for Healthcare Research and Quality, and RTI International, health conditions related to obesity (including type 2 diabetes and heart disease) cost the American health care system over $147 billion each year.
What is this money spent on?

- Open-heart bypass surgery: up to $20,000

- Prescription medication and supplies for diabetes: $115 to $177 monthly–for life

- CPAP machines (to treat sleep apnea): from $150 to $5,000

An obese person costs 42% more to treat than a person of normal weight, which is an additional $1,429. Health insurance plans must pass these costs onto you through higher premiums. In order to recoup these expenses, obese individuals often find it harder to find individual coverage, due to the increased risk of health problems obesity entails.

Pharmaceutical Medication that America's Health System contains has caused many major catastrophes among many civilians health. The Scientists and their laboratories have sent many people spiraling to their death bed due to their synthetic medications and their side effects. The sad part to this is that many people are comfortable with what the doctor prescribe and says what works in fixing their symptoms. The medication prescribed by Doctors most of the time only quiet the symptoms, it does not fix the problem at hand. This is a major problem! Most of the medication issued to patients always causes a side effect or a problem to another organ of the body. But yet many still rely on man's health plan. As a kingdom ambassador, I am so glad that you have this information, this book, to advance you on your path to a healthier you! The scripture tells us "Knowledge shall increase", and because your knowledge has increased in this matter, I pray that you put it to good use. It's the King's will that you be healthy and prosper in EVERY area of your life. You cannot effectively advance the kingdom of G-d sick and depressed! Now is the time for you to change your way of thinking and get motivated to live a healthier lifestyle which doesn't consist of weekly doctor visits, dialysis machines, nightly CPAP ventilation and all other devices used to quiet your symptoms. This day vow that you will make a Kingdom Change, vow that you will live your Kingdom Life as the King ordained from the foundation of the earth. You can do it! Through my publications and product I vow to help you to grow into a clean lifestyle of eating. Believe it or not, I am on the same journey you are on, therefore, we are in this together.

Chapter Five

"Kingdom Foods that heal"

Eliminating unclean foods and eating clean would automatically cleanse your body naturally.

Eating clean will naturally do the following:

1. Perform a bowel cleanse which would eliminate parasites
2. Dental cleanup
3. Cleanse your Kidneys and Lungs
4. Cleanse your liver
5. Cleanse Lymph Nodes
6. Cleanse Your Blood
7. Cleanse your Mind

Because of your body cleansing itself naturally, this would eliminate the big belly syndrome. Your body will begin to eliminate waste at least twice a day. The foods listed in the program below would begin the cleansing process which is a very important piece to the Kingdom health Plan. Proper daily elimination would eliminate body odor, bad breath and acne. As I stated earlier that diseases usually began in the intestines. Therefore, another important piece of the Kingdom Health Plan is body PH. The foods of the bible have healing properties that would eliminate excessive fat and began a healing process within your tabernacle. I want you to know that diseases cannot live in an alkaline body. The body's normal PH is 7.41, anything below a normal body PH of 7.41 is termed acidosis. Anything above the normal body's PH is called alkalosis. To maintain a healthy body, free of disease of any kind, the goal is to maintain a neutral PH of 7.41.

In this chapter I have listed the foods of the biblical scripture and their healing properties that would invite a neutral PH to catapult you on your way to a lifestyle transformation.

Barley – Deuteronomy 8:8

The Bible is filled with reference to barley, which is among the earliest known and most nourishing grains ever to be cultivated. In fact, The Feast of Unleavened Bread was an ancient barley harvest festival that became the celebration of the Passover.

Benefits

Barley improves potency, vigor and strength. It is also recommended as "medicine for the heart." That's because, say nutritionists, it is full of beta glucans – a type of fiber that can lower the risk of heart disease by reducing levels of artery-clogging LDF. A diet that includes lots of barley, three times a day, has lowered blood cholesterol by about 15% in a number of medical studies. That same high fiber content keeps us regular, relieves constipation and wards off a wide variety of digestive problems. It also may help block cancer.

Coriander (Cilantro)

When the Children of Israel wandered in the desert and received manna from the sky, they described it as looking like coriander seed. Ever since, coriander has been called "the healer from heaven." Coriander is an annual plant of the carrot or parsley family and has pink or white flower clusters. The fruit consists of globular, grayish-white colored seeds. It grew wild throughout Egypt, ancient Palestine and other countries in the region. The seeds have pleasant, aromatic oil. They are used as a spice or flavoring for pastries, meats, candies, salads, soups, curries and wine.

Chances are, none of the early peoples suffered from indigestion because coriander has been used for centuries as a treatment for minor stomach ailments. Unlike most medicines for digestive problems, coriander tastes great and has a warm fragrance like citrus and sage.

Benefits
It's recommended for indigestion, flatulence and diarrhea. Externally, it's used to ease muscle and joint pain. Recently, scientists began looking at coriander as an anti-inflammatory treatment for arthritis. Other research has demonstrated that it reduces blood sugar levels, an indication that it may prove to be a useful sugar management tool for diabetics.

Garlic
It's one of the world's oldest healing foods. It was being used both as a favorite food and as a powerful medicine centuries before Moses led the children of Israel out of Egypt and into the wilderness. Garlic was one of the first foods to be deliberately cultivated, although wild varieties grew in abundance.

Evidence of its healing powers is detailed in 4,000 year old records from the ancient kingdom of Sumeria. Depiction of garlic bulbs have been discovered on walls of Egyptian tombs that date back to 3200 B.C. – centuries before Joseph and his brothers settled in Egypt. Before the birth of Christ, the Israelites were using garlic as a major ingredient in their food, as well as a medicine. In fact, they were so fond of garlic and consumed so much of it that in the Mishnah they proudly called themselves "Garlic Eaters".

Benefits
During that same period, ancient records reveal that garlic was the principal ingredient in many remedies that Egyptian healers prescribed as cures for headaches, sore throats and other complaints.

By the time of Moses, garlic was already being used as an anticoagulant, antiseptic, anti-inflammatory and anti-tumor agent, as well as a relief for flatulence, a diuretic, a sedative, a poultice and as a cure for internal parasites.

Garlic may help protect against heart disease and stroke by lowering blood pressure. It contains allylic sulfides, which may neutralize carcinogens. In fact, garlic has been linked to lower rates of stomach cancer too.

Grapes – Numbers 12:23

Grapes were the first things Noah planted after the flood. Grapes were eaten fresh, dried and eaten as raisins just as we do today and pressed into cakes. But most of the crop of the vineyards was made into juice, wine and vinegar.

One reason this delicious fruit was so important in the diet thousands of years ago was because of its high content of boron, a mineral that we now know helps ward off osteoporosis. Boron is now sold as a dietary supplement in health food stores, but the people of the Bible had to get theirs from natural sources. Aside from preventing osteoporosis, grapes offer many healthy benefits.

A cup of raw grapes contain only 58 calories, 0.3 grams of fat; zero cholesterol and vitamins A, B and C. Grapes also contain important minerals such as boron, calcium, potassium and zinc.

Benefits

They fight tooth decay, stop viruses in their tracks and are rich in other ingredients that many researchers believe can head off cancer. Grapes also appear promising as antiviral and antitumor agents.

Leeks

Leeks are also mentioned in the Book of Numbers, as a milder, sweeter version of the onion. In cooking, the leek is extremely versatile when used to flavor other dishes or as a food by itself. It has a more delicate flavor than garlic or onions and forms the basis of many traditional dishes that originated in ancient Israel and neighboring lands. A favorite dish in biblical times – and still popular in present day Middle East – was a kind or porridge made from the white bulb of the leek, rice or similar grains, with crushed almonds and honey added as a sweetener.

Benefits
Leeks were prescribed for infertile women and have traditionally been used internally and externally for a variety of conditions including obesity, kidney complaints, intestinal disorders and coughs

Legumes – 2 Samuel 17:28, 29
As reported in the Book of Samuel, beans were among the highly nutritious foods sent to feed King David's hungry army and restore their strength for the hard times ahead. But how might beans have been so important?

We now know that beans are absolutely packed with soluble fiber, which helps lower LDL and reduces blood pressure. That same fiber also helps keep blood sugar levels stable, staves off hunger and has even been shown to reduce the insulin requirements of people suffering from diabetes. Important as they are to us today, they were even more important as a staple food in biblical times. Beans are a wonderful source of protein as well as being packed full of vitamin C, iron and dietary fiber. In the West, most of us get these either from other foods or from supplements. Unlike our biblical ancestors, today there is a wide range of beans to choose from– red, white and black beans, black-eyed peas or cowpeas, chickpeas, fava, kidney, lentils, lima, split peas, pinto, white, Great Northern, navy and butter beans. All of them offer the same kind of wonderful health benefits.

Benefits
Beans help lower blood pressure and reduce "bad" cholesterol.
Beans also contain chemicals that inhibit the growth of cancer and help control insulin and blood sugar levels so vital to the good health of diabetics. On a more routine level, beans help prevent constipation. They can stop hemorrhoids and other bowel-related problems from developing and help cure them if they do. In those ancient times, beans and garlic were often boiled together, which produced a primitive version of cough medicine that was said to stop even the

most stubborn cough. Beans are also important to diabetics because of their ability to regulate insulin output. Type I diabetes can cut back on their need for insulin by as much as 38% when put on a bean-rich diet. Most of Type II diabetics in the same study were able to stop insulin injections entirely!

Mint

The warm flavor of mint, due to the presence of characteristic essential oils, is well-known to all of us today, just as it was to the Hebrews, Greeks and Romans of Bible times who used mint as medicine as well as a flavoring. Some Bible experts say mint was among the "bitter herbs" of Exodus 12:8 and Numbers 9:11 along with leaves of endive, chicory, lettuce, watercress, sorrel and dandelion, which were eaten as a salad. Mint is one of the "bitter herbs" of the Passover feast today.

Benefits

Modern herbalists recommend peppermint be taken straight or added to foods as a treatment for menstrual cramps, motion and morning sickness, colds and flu, headache and heartburn, fever and insomnia. Medical experts also know that the mints are marvelous for treating dozens of other problems. That's why mints, with their menthol contents, are found in many over the counter remedies for indigestion, minor pain and congestion. The mints are also antispasmodics. They soothe the muscles of the digestive tract and the uterus. But while peppermint may be good for nausea, it may also stimulate menstruation. So doctors war pregnant women to avoid peppermint as a treatment for morning sickness.

Nuts – Song of Songs 6:11

It was no accident that these people of biblical times that included nuts in their diets apparently were not troubled by many of the health disorders that seem to plague us in these modern times such as heart disease, cancer and diabetes. The belief that nuts were a powerful healing food continued into the Middle Ages. Walnuts were considered so powerful that they were included in a prescription to ward off even the dreaded Black Plague that swept Europe throughout the Middle Ages.

Benefits

We now know that nuts contain the right mixtures of natural ingredients whose benefits include cancer prevention, a lower risk of heart disease and help for diabetics. The oil found in walnuts is considered healthful because it is one of these "good guy" polyunsaturated fats and tends to lower blood cholesterol levels. Nuts are just as much a part of the daily life and diet today in the countries surrounding the Mediterranean as they were in biblical times when Jacob instructed Judah to send them as a gift to Joseph, the governor of Egypt.

Olives

The olive was certainly one of the most valuable and versatile tress of biblical times. It is mentioned frequently throughout the Bible. Probably the most famous reference to olive oil and its healing powers is in the parable of the Good Samaritan, in which the Samaritan cares for a beaten and robbed traveler, treating his wounds with oil and wine. Olive oil is a high-energy food and one of the most digestible of all fats. The ancients of biblical times found ways to incorporate it in many of these meals. The "anointing with oil" that was a sacred tradition among biblical people was probably done with olive oil. One ancient piece of folk wisdom tells us that "olive oil makes all your aches and pains go away."

Benefits

It was used to maintain the suppleness of skin and muscle, to heal abrasions and to soothe the burning and drying effects of the sun and wind. Pliny and Hippocrates, the noted physicians of ancient Greece prescribed medicines containing olive oil and olive leaves as cures for such disorders as inflammation of the gums, insomnia, nausea and boils In countries with the highest rate of cardiovascular diseases, diets were heavy in saturated fats, which increased cholesterol levels. The saturated fatty acids are found in animal fats, such as butter and lard. Monounsaturated fatty acids do not have cholesterol. Olive oil contains 56-83 percent of these acids, also called oleic acids. Olive oil is rich in monounsaturated fats, which may lower blood cholesterol. Eating four or five tablespoons of olive oil daily dramatically improves the blood profiles of heart attack patients. And 2/3 of a tablespoon daily lowered blood pressure in men. If you're trying to reduce the amount of fat in your diet to avoid the risk of heart attack, think of olive oil as an ideal replacement.

Onions – Numbers 11:5

Like its cousin, garlic, the onion is noted as a cure-all. And the folk healers hold it in high regard as far back as 6,000 years ago or more. Although onion was only mentioned once in the Bible, it was within a list of foods with the best healing properties. Hence, its inclusion here. Onions were considered such an important source of energy and endurance, wrote Herodotus, the Greek historian, that the Egyptian pharaohs spent nine tons of gold for onions to feed the slaves and laborers who built the pyramids. Whether of not it was an acquired taste history doesn't say. But the Jews took a distinct fondness for the onion when they followed Moses into the wilderness

Benefits

So at least 3,000 years before the birth of Christ, onions were treasured both as food and for their therapeutic value – particularly in the treatment of kidney and bladder problems. Onions have been used externally as an antiseptic and a pain reliever. They've been taken internally as a tonic to soothe intestinal gas pains and to alleviate the symptoms of hypertension, high blood sugar and elevated cholesterol. It's said the fold remedies in many other cultures called for the juice of an onion and syrup made from honey to treat coughs, colds and asthma attacks. A tonic of onions prescribed for kidney stones and to eliminate excessive fluids. Modern herbalists recommend onion syrup as an expectorant (it helps eliminate mucus from the respiratory tract). Onions are also believed to be diuretic and to reduce high blood pressure.

Wheat – Jeremiah 41:8

For the people of the Bible, wheat was a great food treasure. It was a staple at most every meal. In addition, wheat could make the difference between life and death because of its nutritional value and the protection it offered against a host of disabling, often deadly, disorders and diseases. Wheat was the "staff of life." Because it was such an important part of everyday survival it became an important religious symbol for both Jews and Christians. An abundant harvest was a blessing from God. Biblical people ate their grain boiled and parched, soaked and roasted, and even ate it green from the stalk. It was pounded, dried or crushed to be baked into casseroles, porridges, soups, parched grain salads and desserts such as puddings and flans. Bible scholars say that Ezekiel's Bread was intended to be a survival food during the dark days of the Babylonian conquest because it contains wheat, barley, beans, lentils, millet and spelt. The Israelites put their faith in this multigrain foodstuff to maintain their health and stay fighting fit.

Much of the wheat the Israelites ate was actually the wheat bran, the outermost layers of the wheat kernel which is nearly all fiber.

Benefits

It is now well-established just how critical fiber is to healthy digestion and efficient bowel function. Wheat bran is also absolutely loaded with crucial B vitamins and protein. Wheat germ ranks up there for its all-encompassing nutritional value. A ¼ cup packs 5 grams of fiber, as well as B vitamins, iron, magnesium and zinc. It's also rich in chromium, manganese and vitamin E. Whole wheat bread contains triple the fiber found in white bread and is much richer in magnesium and vitamin B. Wheat bran's high fiber content is one of the richest dietary sources of insoluble fiber known. Nothing quite matches the power of this fiber in keeping wastes moving regularly throughout our systems. The fiber in wheat is our best protection against – and cure of – constipation. It prevents intestinal infections, hemorrhoids, varicose veins, improves bowel function, and guards us against colon cancer.

I am a firm believer that eating, "Tahor" which is a Hebrew word for clean, would erase stubborn fat and eliminate dreadful disease within our bodies. It's not by accident that the most high gave the children of Israel dietary laws to adhere to. Going outside of eating clean can and will cause us to age a lot quicker than usual, cause fatique, headaches and all other negative things that associate with unclean eating. I challenge all of you to implement the Kingdom Health Plan in your lifestyle. Exercise daily, even if it's just a short walk around the neighborhood, exercise is also part of his health plan. He wants us to live our life in obedience in all things. As we do this, we would see his kingdom manifested here on earth, as it is in heaven.

Chapter Six

What is Imperial 120 day Alkaline Plan?

The Alkaline 120 day plan is a health strategy of the Imperial Nation health system. The Plan is based around the idea that the foods you eat can alter the acidity or alkalinity (the pH value) of your body. Let me explain how that works…

When you metabolize foods and extract the energy (calories) from them, you are actually burning the foods, except that it happens in a slow and controlled fashion.

When you burn foods, they actually leave an ash residue, just like when you burn wood in a furnace.

As it turns out, this ash can be acidic or alkaline (or neutral)… and proponents of this 120 day plan can **directly** affect the acidity of your body.

So if you eat foods that are acidic, it makes your body acidic. If you eat foods that are alkaline, it makes your body alkaline. Neutral foods has no effect. Simple.

Acidic food is thought to make you vulnerable to illness and disease, whereas alkaline food is considered protective. By choosing more alkaline foods, you should be able to "alkalize" your body and improve your health.

Why do Imperial Nation have it's own health system in place?

If you were go and research the stats, you will find that majority of civilians die at the discretion of the pharmaceutical and medical field. Many die to medical error.

Medical errors persist as the No. 3 killer in the U.S. – third only to heart disease and cancer – claiming the lives of some 400,000 people each year.

When we enroll in a Medical System, we are enrolling or signing our name on a contract which give this system the right to do what they want to do to us and our children. You must understand that the pills prescribed only suppresses the systems. It does not heal the underlining or the root cause. Therefore, we continue to get sicker over a period of time. Imperial Health System deal with the root of all disease.

Our health System is based on an Alkaline Structure. Our mission and goal is to balance the body ph, In order to obtain a healthy state, our 120 day Alkaline Plan is structured to do just that. You must carefully follow the plan in order to obtain the maximum results.

Before getting started on this 120 day journey, make sure that you have taken the first step of the process, which is the PH Assessment.

Why 120 Days? We believe that all bad habits can be broken in 21 days, some may require a longer time in order to get in the flow of a healthier lifestyle. With intensed research also with having a background in Respiratory Therapy, I know that the body can heal it self. Our 120 day plan will jump start you on the right path of living a disease free lifestyle.

Getting started on this journey requires making sure that you have the foods needed.

Below is the list of Alkaline and Acidic Foods. Please base your Alkaline diet on the Alkaline Foods list. The other 2 list are foods to stay away from during these 120 days.

Alkaline Diet Health Tips

Alkaline Foods

Grains, Cereals & Breads
- Amaranth
- Buckwheat
- Kamut
- Millet
- Quinoa
- Spelt
- Sprouted Breads
- Sprouted Tortillas
- Yeast-Free Breads

Sweets & Desserts
- None

Beans & Legumes
- All moderately acidic

Nuts & Seeds
- Almond Butter
- Almonds
- Carraway Seeds
- Cumin Seeds
- Fennel Seeds
- Hemp Seeds
- Pumpkin Seeds
- Sesame Seeds
- Sunflower Seeds

Drinks
- Alkaline Water
- Barley Grass
- Huide
- Coconut Water
- Fresh Lemon & Lime Water
- Fresh Veg Juices
- Green Drinks
- Green Tea
- Herbal Tea
- Wheat Grass Juice
- Udo's Choice
- Beyond Greens

Diary & Meat
- None

Condiments & Spices
- (Unfermented Soy)
- Almond Butter
- Bee Pollen
- Bragg Aminos
- Chili Pepper
- Cinnamon
- Curry Powders
- Ginger
- Guacamole (fresh made)
- Herbs (all)
- Houmous
- Lemon Juice
- Lime Juice
- Sea Salt

Oriental Vegetables
- Daikon
- Dandelion Root
- Kombu
- Maitake
- Nori
- Reishi
- Sea Vegetables
- Shitake
- Umeboshi
- Wakame

Debatable / Moderately Acidic Foods

Grains, Cereals & Breads
- Brown Rice

Sweets & Desserts
- Lo Han Guo
- Stevia

Beans & Legumes
- (Chick Peas)
- Black Beans
- Canned Beans
- Garbanzo Beans
- Kidney Beans
- Lentils
- Lima Beans
- Mung Beans
- Navy Beans
- Pinto Beans
- Red Beans
- Soy Beans
- White Beans

Nuts & Seeds
- Brazil Nuts
- Cashews
- Hazel Nuts
- Peanut Butter
- Peanuts
- Walnuts

Drinks
- Tap, Bottled & Unfiltered Water
- Pasteurised Tomato Juice

Diary & Meat
- Butter (Raw)
- Buttermilk (Raw)
- Cheese (Raw)
- Milk (Raw)
- Quorn
- Tofu
- Whey (Raw)
- Yogurt (Organic Fresh)

Condiments & Spices
- Apple Cider Vinegar
- Miso
- Tahini

Acidic Foods

Grains, Cereals & Breads
- Barley
- Bran, oat
- Bran, wheat
- Bread
- Corn
- Corn Chips
- Cornstarch
- Crackers
- Flour
- Flour
- Granola
- Macaroni
- Noodles
- Oatmeal
- Oats (rolled)
- Pasta
- Processed Grains
- Rice Cakes
- Rye
- Spaghetti
- Wheat Germ
- White Rice
- Wheat

Sweets & Desserts
- ALL Sugar, Sugar Products & Artificial Sweeteners

Beans & Legumes
- All moderately acidic

Nuts & Seeds
- All moderately acidic

Drinks
- Alcohol
- Black Tea
- Cocoa
- Coffee
- Energy Drinks
- Milk
- Pasteurized Juice
- Soda

Dairy & Meat
- ALL products

Condiments & Spices
- Fermented Sauces
- Jams & Preserves
- Mayonnaise
- Soy Sauce
- Sweet Chilli Sauce
- Tomato Ketchup
- Vinegar

The Imperial Kingdom Health Plan

Products Needed for the 120 Day Journey

Alkaline H20-One Gallon (providing that you bring your jugs, 7 gallons of water per week will be $50.00 per month while doing the 120 day plan or if you are on the pledge system your water is free. If Imperial have to provide the jugs, the cost will be $70.00 per month.) Please note that we will fill one weeks worth at a time.

Imperial Alkaline Supreme-One Teaspoon 3 times a day

Imperial Tonic-One Teaspoon 3 times a day

Outer Hygeine:

Imperial Deodorant

Imperial Tooth Paste

Imperial Natural Bath Wash/Soap

Imperial Natural Shampoo & Conditioner

Start your morning with any of the following Alkaline Items:

Alkaline Green Smoothie

Recipe 1:

3/4 cup raw coconut water or filtered water

- 1/2 cup raw coconut meat or 1 tablespoon raw creamed coconut
- 2 cups spinach
- 1 medium avocado, peeled and pitted
- 1/2 medium cucumber, chopped
- 2 teaspoons finely grated lime zest
- 2 limes, peeled and halved
- 20 drops alcohol-free liquid stevia
- pinch Celtic sea salt
- 1 teaspoon minced ginger (optional)
- 1 1/2 cups ice, plus more if needed

1. Throw all of your ingredients in your Blender and blast on high for 30 to 60 seconds until smooth and creamy.
2. Makes two 16-ounce glasses.

Recipe 2:

Avocado –1 Peeled,

Chopped Spinach or Baby Greens

1 Large Handful Cucumber

½ Whole, Chopped Vine Tomatoes

2 Chopped Red Pepper

½ Chopped Celery

1 Stick, Chopped Udo's Choice Green Blend

1 Tablespoon Water Optionally Added To Thin

Recipe 3:

Mixed Sprouts (Alfalfa, Broccoli, Chick Pea etc)

2 Cups Spinach or Baby Greens

1 Large Handful Cucumber

2 Inch Slice, Chopped Water – 1 Small Cup (100ml-200ml)

Recipe 4:

Spinach or Baby Greens

2 Large Handfuls Apple

1 Chopped Cucumber

1 Medium, Chopped Parsley

½ Small Cup Celery

1 Stick, Chopped Lemon

1 Squeezed Ginger

1 Small Piece, Peeled & Chopped Water

1 Small Cup (100ml-200ml)

Recipe 5:

Avocado

1 Peeled, Chopped Sprouted Peas

2 Cups Spinach or Baby Greens

1 Large Handful Sugar Snap Peas

1 Cup Apple

1 Small, Chopped Cayenne Pepper

Pinch Sea Salt Pinch Water – 1 Cup (200ml)

Recipe 6

Avocado – 1 Peeled,

Chopped Kale - 1 Large Handful Lime

½ Squeezed Lemon – ½ Squeezed Banana

1 Peeled & Chopped Mixed Seeds – 2 Tablespoons (Chopped)

Apple Juice – 1 Small Cup (100-200ml)

Water – Optionally Added To Thin Consistency

Wheatgrass Powder – 1 Teaspoon (Optional)

LUNCH RECIPES TO CHOOSE FROM:

"Creamy Avocado-Broccoli Soup"

Ingredients for 4 Servings
2-3 flowers broccoli
1 small avocado
1 yellow onion
1 green or red pepper
1 celery stalk
2 cups vegetable broth (yeast-free)
Celtic Sea Salt to taste
Some cumin, basil, fresh cilantro or your favorite spices to taste

Fresh Garden Vegetable Soup

2 large carrots
1 small zucchini
1 celery stalk
1 cup of broccoli
3 stalks of asparagus
1 yellow onion
1 quart of (<u>alkaline</u>) water
4-5 tsps of yeast-free vegetable broth
1 tsps fresh basil
2 tsps sea salt to taste

Alkaline Broccoli Salad with Tofu

Ingredients for 2 servings
300g organic tofu
2 flowers of broccoli
5 tbsp. cold pressed olive oil
2 tbsp. soy sauce
1 tbsp. fresh lemon juice
Some sea salt and pepper to taste
1 garlic clove
½ red pepper bell for garnishing

Put diced tofu with some oil in a pan and fry for around 15 minutes. Turn off the stove, pour the soy sauce over the tofu and set aside. Now stir-fry the broccoli for 10 minutes. Also set aside to cool off.

For the dressing, put the olive oil, the fresh lime juice, salt, pepper and the garlic in a blender and mix well until smooth. Then, put the tofu and the broccoli in a bowl, pour over the dressing and mix well.

References
The daily green article
Summer tomato article
Naturodoc.com
Whitedovebooks
Truth Publishing

Imperial Nation Publishing
Dallas, Tx 75150